Naturopathy:

Easy Guide How To Stay Healthy Without Pills

Table of Contents

Introduction

Are you tired of taking all those biochemical pills to rectify several issues related to your health? If your answer is "yes", then you are ready to take the first step towards a healthier future.

We all know that most of these new-age drugs have numerous side effects on our body. These biochemical drugs that we all consume can compromise with our body in more ways than we can imagine. From causing a neurological effect to tampering our core genetics – the list goes on and on.

Not just that, most of these modern treatments cost a fortune. In today's world, it is can get quite tough to spend such a large sum of money on pills or any other mainstream medical treatment.

To overcome these problems, you can always take the assistance of various alternative medical treatments. Over the course of time, medical science has developed in various other aspects as well. Naturopathy, Ayurveda, Homeopathy, Yoga, etc. are some other popular ways to treat several physical or mental problems related to your body.

In this guide, we will make you familiar with some of the most popular naturopathy and alternative medicine treatments for various common issues. Read on and be ready to ditch all those mainstream medical treatments. Start living your life without any pills and enjoy it to the fullest.

Chapter 1 – An Introduction To Naturopathy

Naturopathy is a branch of alternative medicine that deals with various pseudo-scientific principles. Instead of relying on any aggressive allopathic treatment, various non-invasive and natural treatments are practiced to fight an illness.

The concept of self-healing is largely associated with naturopathy, which makes it so different from any conventional allopathic treatment. The assistance of natural and self-healing treatment is taken instead of various evidence-based medicines (pills).

The modern concept of naturopathy has been evolved from Greece. Though, its roots can be linked to the ancient civilizations of India and China as well. It is a wide concept and comprises of various other age-old practices of Ayurveda, homeopathy, Unani, yoga, and more.

Various popular alternative medical treatments have certainly evolved over the last few decades. There are dedicated courses for alternative medicine that are practiced all over the world. In a few countries, naturopathy is considered as vital as any other leading allopathic treatment.

In this guide, we will make you familiar with various home remedies that can make your life a whole lot better. With the help of naturopathy and other alternative medical practices, you can easily treat mild problems like a headache, bad stomach, cold, bad throat, etc.

Though, there are lots of alternative medical practices that are considered even more powerful than modern science and can treat dreadful diseases like cancer as well. Before we discuss various remedies, it is important to know why you should prefer alternative medicine over allopathic treatments.

Benefits of alternative medicine

Alternative medicine (including naturopathy) has plenty of benefits. We have listed only a handful of them, so that you can get an idea about it before practicing it on your own.

No side-effect: This is one of the most evident benefits of naturopathy. Unlike any allopathic treatment, it doesn't cause any adverse side-effect on your body.

No addiction: It has been observed that people easily get addicted to pills and other commonly found mainstream remedies. Needless to say, it can have an adverse effect on your body. This is definitely not the same with most of the alternative medical treatments.

Low cost: We all know how costly mainstream treatments can be at times. If you don't have a health insurance, then covering your medical bills can be a herculean task. Additionally, even insurance doesn't cover every medical bill at times. Naturopathy, on the other hand, is quite cheap and has plenty of homemade remedies that won't cost you a dime.

Mental peace: After practicing these alternative medical practices, you can see a drastic difference in your life. Not just physical, they can also heal your mental scars. For instance, yoga and meditation can help you attain the kind of mental peace that no other mainstream treatment can provide.

Painless treatment: While a surgery or a complex procedure might cause a lot of pain in your body, the same is not true for naturopathy. Most of these alternative treatments are quite painless in nature and provide fruitful results.

Targets the whole body: Unlike allopathic treatments (which targets only a specific body part), naturopathy works on your whole body. It helps in cleaning your entire body – from head to toe without injecting any harmful products.

Reliable: This might surprise you, but there are a few naturopathy and alternative medical practices that are considered more reliable than the new-age aggressive techniques. For instance, Ayurveda is more than 5000 years old. Its first recorded surgery (removal of cataract) took place in the 5th century BC.

Long-term effect: While after taking pills, you might feel relaxed, it can't provide a permanent solution for you. On the other hand, natural therapy might take a while, but will work on the root of the problem to provide a long-term effect.

Before you proceed

After getting to know about all the amazing benefits of alternative medicine, you must be excited to dive in and start treating your body as a temple. Nevertheless, before you proceed, it is important that you are aware of the common malpractices that exist in today's world related to alternative medicine.

Limited knowledge: When it comes to alternative medicine, you can't put a substitute just like that. It is of vital importance that you do your bit of research before proceeding.

Impure products: If you live in a city or are buying products online (or from a nearby store), chances are that you might get an impure or adulterated product. Before you make any purchase, make sure that all these products are pure and naturally harvested.

Wrong marketing: These days, alternative medicine is marketed in a wrong way. Don't dive into it as a tourist. Most of these practices might take more time than any invasive procedure, but it will certainly be worth it in the long run.

So what are you waiting for? Step into a new world of naturopathy and alternative medicine with us while having an open perspective.

Chapter 2 – Natural Homemade Remedies

It has been discovered that most of the times we suffer from common illnesses like a headache or joint pain. Instead of simply relying on pills and attaining a temporary relief, go for these natural remedies to work on the root of your problem.

We have listed various homemade natural remedies for different problems that will certainly come handy to you on numerous occasions.

Headaches and Migraines

In this fast-paced world, lots of people suffer from persisting headaches. It has also been observed that millions of people out there suffer from a regular migraine pain as well. Most of the mainstream medicines might not work to control your migraine or headache pain. Ditch those biochemical headache pills and give these natural treatments a try.

Ginger

It has been proved that ginger can improve the quality of your blood vessels, providing more oxygen to your head.

To start with, mix ginger juice with lemon juice and consume it twice a day.

If the headache is severe, then make a ginger paste (one teaspoon of ginger powder with two tablespoons of water) and gradually rub it on your temple region.

You can always chew a few pieces of ginger or inhale its vapor (by boiling water and putting a piece of ginger or its powder in it).

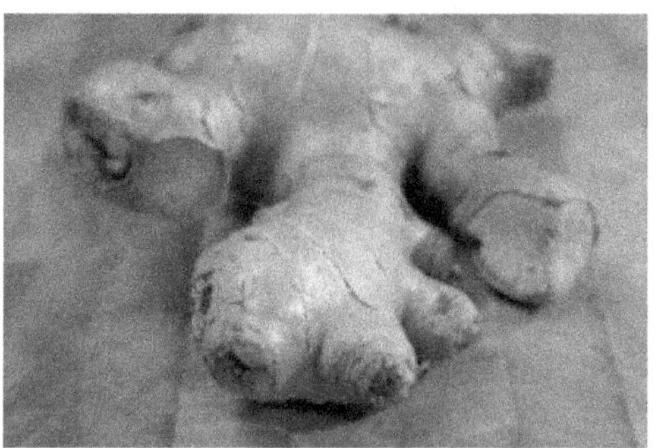

Lavender oil

It is an excellent remedy to treat headaches instantly. Though, you should apply lavender oil carefully (it should not be consumed orally).

Just take a few droplets of lavender oil and apply it gently on your head. If the headache is quite persisting, then add a few drops of lavender oil in boiling water and inhale its vapor.

Mint Juice

Not only refreshing, mint juice is also quite effective for a migraine. It has menthol content in it that can provide an instant relief to headaches. You can also consume it in an old-fashioned way or simply rub its leaves on your forehead as well.

Mint tea is another great alternative to cure headache related to tension and stress. You can also add a few coriander leaves in it to maximize its impact.

Peppermint oil

If the headache is caused by tension, then peppermint oil can work wonders for you. Consume it the same way as lavender oil to get productive results. It can also treat sinus and widen your blood vessels to maximize your brain's oxygen intake.

Basil

Basil can relax your muscles and provide long-term relief related to your migraine or headache pain. It also provides a calming effect to our body and can help you overcome tension or stress as well.

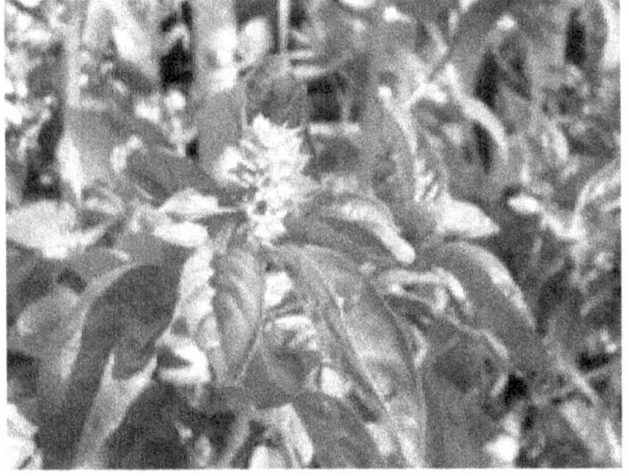

Take 4-5 leaves of basil and put them in boiling water. Let them simmer for a while. Now, put the leaves in your tea (with some honey, if needed) and drink it when hot.

If you can't drink it, then you can always put a few leaves in boiling water and inhale the vapor as well.

If you can, then simply chew a few basil leaves to get immediate results.

Additionally, you can do it in an old-fashioned way and rub a few leaves on your forehead/temple region by mixing it with oil.

With the unpredicted change in weather, it is quite common to suffer from a sore throat or cough these days. Instead of weakening your immune system, take the assistance of these natural remedies.

Licorice root

It has been proven scientifically that licorice root can drastically diminish cough and heal a sore throat. You can take its small slice and place it in your mouth (without chewing it), letting its extract soothe your throat. Additionally, you can mix it with hot water and create a gargle solution as well.

Honey

Honey mixed with tea is the perfect household remedy for a bad throat. Honey is quite effective for nighttime coughs in particular. It has amazing healing properties and can work wonders at times. You can consume honey with some green tea to soothe your bad throat.

Marshmallow root

This might surprise you, but marshmallow root can provide an instant remedy to your sore throat. It has mucus-like particles that can add a special coating to your throat and prevent it from any damage.

Just add a few pieces of it in boiling water (with a few added herbs, if needed) to make an aromatic tea. Sip this hot tea 2-3 times a day to get an instant relief.

Slippery elm

Just like marshmallow root, slippery elm also has the same mucus-like substance that can provide an added layer to your throat. It can soothe your throat instantly while absorbing the cough.

Just mix it with water to create a gel-like mixture. Use boiling water while preparing this mixture and take small sips of it. Drink it 2-3 times a day to get a proper cure for your bad throat.

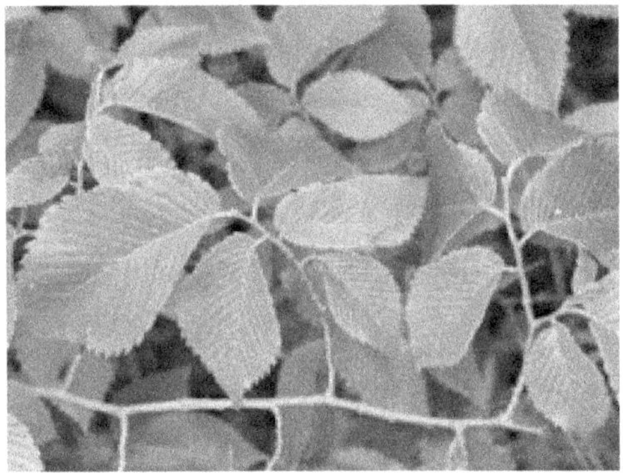

Garlic

This might surprise you, but garlic has plenty of medicinal properties and can help you strengthen your immunity as well. If you are having a bad throat, then take one clove of garlic and slice it in half.

Now, place it in your mouth and instead of taking a bite, prefer sucking it. Just take small bites from its corner at regular intervals. This will release a substance, known as *allicin* into your mouth. This can cure your sore throat instantaneously.

Chamomile tea

This is probably one of the oldest remedies for a sore throat. Chamomile has excellent antioxidant, astringent and anti-inflammatory property, which makes it a must-have herb for every household.

It has been found that Chamomile tea can help one fight cough and sore throat to a great extent. Its regular consumption can also strengthen your immune system.

Gargles

If nothing else works, then follow this age-old home remedy and provide a warm and soothing effect to your throat. Not only it breaks secretions, but also kills bacteria to heal your throat.

Take a half teaspoon of regular salt and add it to a glass of warm water. If your throat is swollen, then prefer gargling with warm salt water in every 3-4 hours.

Additionally, to maximize its impact, you can add a pinch of baking soda in the solution as well. It will kill any other kind of fungi growth and provide a soothing effect to your throat.

Seasonal Allergies

Who doesn't suffer from seasonal allergies, right? Though, we resist taking all those anti-allergic pills many times since they make us feel sleepy and drowsy all day long. Take the assistance of these natural remedies and stay at the top of your game all day long without any unwanted seasonal allergy.

Apple cider vinegar

This age-old technique can help you overcome any allergic reaction in no time. It can reduce mucous production and strengthen your immune system as well. To start with, just take a teaspoon of organic apple cider vinegar and mix it with a glass of water.

Make sure that you don't take it directly. It is recommended to dilute it in water for an ideal usage. You can initially take it twice a day to fight your allergic reaction.

Nettle Peppermint tea

Nettle is one of the most incredible herbs of all and can be used to cure a persisting allergy. It can also regulate your blood pressure and cure joint pain as well. Combine it with peppermint to create highly-beneficial remedies. It has anti-inflammatory property and can make you stay comfortable all day long.

To make nettle peppermint tea, take either dried powdered material or fresh ones. We recommend taking freshly chopped leaves of peppermint and nettle leaf. If you don't have them, then go for their powders. Mix them with warm water and a few drops of honey and lemon.

You need to boil this mixture for 5-10 minutes before taking its sip. Drink it twice a day to get immediate relief.

Citrus drinks

Vitamin C is widely known to cure seasonal allergies. It can readily be found in citrus fruits like lemon or orange. Take 2 oranges and half lemon in order to prepare a fresh glass of juice. Add some honey and a pinch of salt before drinking it. You can do this 2-3 times a day. Not only will it cure your allergic reaction, but will also keep you hydrated all day long.

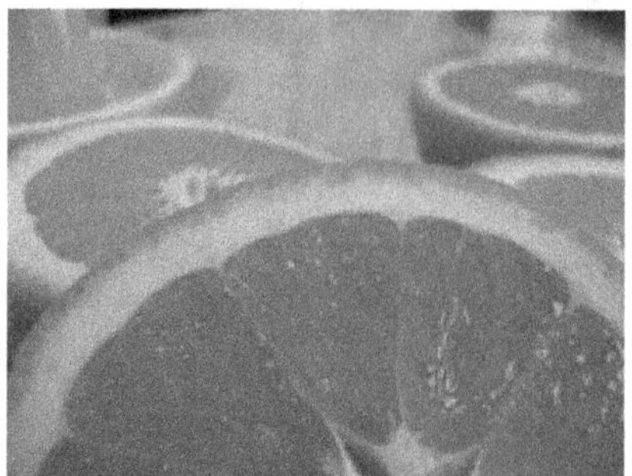

Red onion water

Red onion has a natural substance, *quercetin,* which can help your body fight an allergic reaction easily. It can widen your airways and prevent the blocking of your windpipe, so that you can breathe without any trouble.

To start with, take one medium-sized red onion and slice it. Pour it in different cups of water and add a few drops of honey. Now, let it infuse for the next 10-12 hours at least. When it is done, drink the water 2-3 times a day. You can just keep the mixture in the fridge and drink it for the next 3-4 days.

Dandruff and Scalp Issues

It is high-time when you get rid of all those anti-dandruff shampoos. Most of these products have harmful chemicals and can cause an adverse effect to your scalp. It can often lead to hair fall. Take the help of these natural ingredients to get rid of dandruff permanently.

Acacia concinna and Curd

This is undoubtedly the best solution to get rid of dandruff. Take *Acacia concinna* powder and mix it with a half cup of curd. Add a few drops of lemon juice and coconut oil in the mixture. Now, apply this mixture on your scalp and let it rest for the next 15-20 minutes. Simply wash it away to get stronger hair.

Coconut oil and Lemon

You might already know how beneficial coconut oil is for our scalp. This home remedy won't cost you much as well and will let you get rid of unwanted dandruff in no time. Initially, heat two tablespoons of coconut oil and add another tablespoon of lemon juice in the mixture. Massage this mixture on your scalp gently and let it rest for another 30 minutes or so before washing it off with shampoo.

Fenugreek Pack

For years, people have been using Fenugreek seeds to get rid of dandruff. To start with, soak Fenugreek seed in water for 10-12 hours (overnight). Drain out the mixture and mash the seeds. This will result into a paste. Apply it on your scalp and let it rest for an hour before washing it off.

Tea Tree Oil

Tea Tree has plenty of benefits and should be present in every house. It can provide visible results while getting rid of dandruff as well. Just pour a few drops of tea tree oil on your scalp and massage it for the next 10-15 minutes. Afterward, simply wash it off with an herbal shampoo.

From sunburn to those unwanted blisters, your skin can get damaged in different ways. Though we will cover various techniques to cure dry skin and rashes as well in this guide, it is also important to know how to treat a skin burn or blister beforehand.

Aloe Vera

It is considered as a natural cure for burns and other skin-related injuries like blisters. It has amazing healing properties and hydrates the skin. Simply peel and cut a leaf of aloe vera and take out its gel. Now, gently apply this gel on your skin and let it heal your blisters. If you don't have any aloe vera plant, then you can always buy its gel from the market.

Turmeric

Turmeric has highly-beneficial antiseptic properties and can heal your skin from sunburn or blisters. To start with, take a tablespoon of turmeric powder and mix it with water to form a paste. Gently rub it on your skin and let it dry. To maximize its effect, you can always mix turmeric powder with curd and add barley to the mixture as well. Let it rest for an hour before washing it gently with cold water.

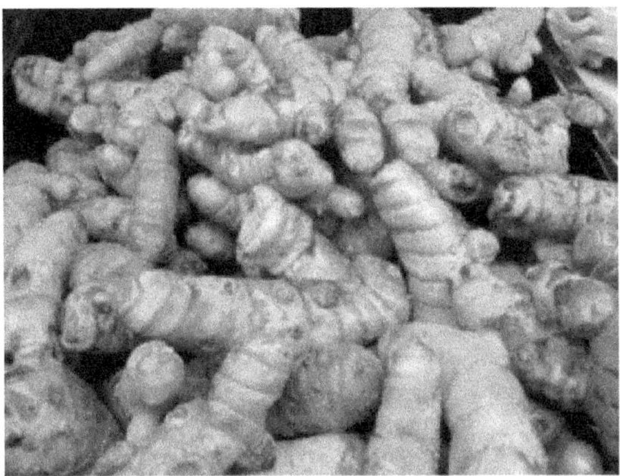

Oatmeal

Oatmeal is extremely healthy for your skin and can heal burns pretty fast. You can always take an oatmeal bath to cleanse your skin as well. Simply fill your bathtub with water and two cups of powdered oatmeal. Treat your body with it for an hour or so.

Also, you can wrap a cup of oatmeal in a muslin cloth and boil it for a few minutes in water. Now, allow it to cool and use it as a sponge to heal your burns.

Vomiting and Diarrhea

Having a bad stomach? Don't worry! You no longer need to take all those pills and wait for them to work against the odds. When it comes to a bad stomach, natural remedies can work instantly. Give these options a try and say goodbye to problems like diarrhea or bad motion.

Black tea

It is considered as one of the best treatments for diarrhea. Just add a little cream or milk to your tea and sip it when it is still hot. Do it twice a day to get a stable stomach.

Yogurt

If you are having severe vomiting, then you should definitely consider consuming yogurt 2-3 times a day. It has natural bacteria that help in digestion and will provide a cooling effect to your stomach. You can also add cumin seeds and fenugreek seeds in yogurt and mix it finely to prepare a solution. This will lead to a better digestion of other substances as well.

Goldenseal

Goldenseal provides an excellent digestive aid and kills all the unwanted bacteria in your system. Just consume a tablespoon of dry Goldenseal powder with warm water and get instant relief from diarrhea.

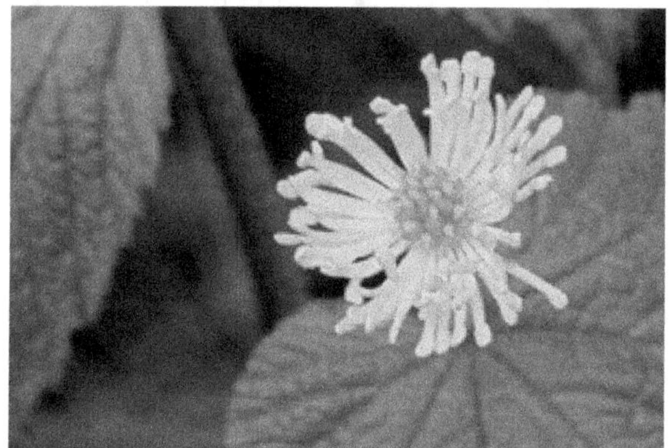

Lemon, Ginger (and Black Pepper) Mix

If you are not feeling good or having vomits, then you should definitely try this solution. Take a tablespoon of lemon juice and add a small teaspoon of ginger paste to it. Sprinkle it with black pepper and mix the solution. Take this 2-3 times a day to get instant relief.

Cold and Flu

Whenever we get cold or a bad flu, we often take the assistance of pills. Though, nothing really works out and we undergo a torture of a running nose for 3-5 days. You might have heard people saying that there is no ideal treatment for flu and that it has to run a whole cycle.

Well, they are wrong. There might be no ideal allopathic treatment for cold, but there are plenty of ways to fight it with natural aids. Here are some foolproof homemade remedies for cold and flu.

Garlic, Lemon, and Honey Mix

This is undoubtedly one of the best ways to beat cold. For years people have been using this age-old technique and it never ceases to disappoint them. To start with, take a small clove of garlic and crush it. Place it in a cup and add 3-4 tablespoons of lemon juice to it. Add a few drops of honey into the mix to make it sweet. Simply consume it a few times to cure your flu.

Coconut Oil and Peppermint Rub

If your flu is quite aggressive, then you should definitely make this all-natural vapor rub. Peppermint has menthol and when combined with coconut oil, it can be used in different ways. To make this rub, take ¼ cup of coconut oil and add 5-6 drops of peppermint essential oil to it. Stir the mixture and keep it in an airtight container. Simply rub it on your chest, palms, neck, or any other body part before going to bed.

Echinacea

For over 400 years, Native Americans have been using Echinacea to treat flu and cold. It has amazing medicinal properties and can be used to strengthen our immune system. It has been scientifically proven that Echinacea can reduce the effect of the common cold by 50%.

In order to consume it, just take a few grams of Echinacea powder (made of its roots, stems, and leaves) and prepare its tea by mixing it with hot water. Consume it 2-3 times a day to get immediate relief from cold.

Elderberry

Yes, this might surprise you, but those delicious elderberries are known to kill virus for ages. If there are no raw elderberries nearby, then just buy its tincture and take a few droplets of it (with water) 3-4 times a day. You will start feeling better in no time.

Horseradish and Ginger Root mix

Both horseradish and ginger root has antiseptic properties and can strengthen your immune system. Shred them down and mix it with boiling water to prepare its tea. You can also consume them in their raw form (in small quantity). Consume it multiple times a day to get desirable results.

Sore Muscles, Arthritis, and Joint Pain

It doesn't matter if you are experiencing joint pain out of aging, if you are recovering from an injury, or if you simply had a bad day – we all experience pain in our muscles and joints way too often. Though, it mostly happens due to deficiency of vitamins and vital minerals (like iron and magnesium) in our body.

Instead of simply taking their substitutes, why not take the assistance of a natural remedy and cure your arthritis, muscle, and joint pain.

Dandelion leaves

They are rich in vitamin A and C, and can heal your muscles and bones in no time. You can either take a teaspoon of dried powdered leaves or simply crush a few fresh leaves as well. Mix it with boiling water and consume it twice a day. If you find it bitter, then simply mix it with virgin oil and massage it on your skin 3-4 times a day.

White Willow Tea

It is known as the original aspirin and was used as a painkiller in the 5th century BC as well. Either take a bark of white willow (and shred it) or take a teaspoon of its powder form. Now, mix it with boiling water and add a few drops of lemon juice and honey to the solution. Drink this tea 2-3 times a day to get relief from your pain.

Peppermint and Eucalyptus Oil

Eucalyptus is widely known to provide a relief to arthritis. It also has pain-relieving properties and will keep you at ease for sure. To start with, take 5-6 drops of both, peppermint and eucalyptus oil. Now, add 2 tablespoons of any other carrier oil (almond or olive oil) in the mixture and store it in a dark airtight bottle. Apply the mixture gently on your bones or joints to kill the pain.

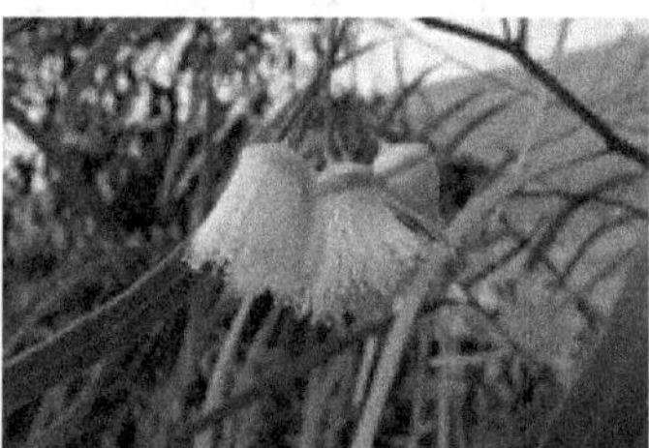

Juniper Berry Tea

A latest research has found several medicinal properties in juniper. It has a substance known as *terpinen*, which can cure arthritis in less time. Though, before you proceed, you should note that juniper should not be consumed if you are pregnant. To start with, take a teaspoon of dried juniper berries and mix it with boiling water. Let the mixture boil for 15-20 minutes before adding a few drops of honey. Drink this tea 2-3 times a day.

Cayenne pepper mix

If you are suffering from rheumatoid arthritis, then you can't find a better solution than this. You can either get a readily available cayenne pepper ointment from the market or prepare one yourself by mixing it with oil. Apply it on your skin a few times a day and say goodbye to your arthritis pain.

Ginger and Turmeric Tea

For years, ginger and turmeric tea are considered as the first choice to provide relief to sore muscles and body pain. Simply take 2 cups of water, a teaspoon of ginger powder, and a teaspoon of turmeric powder. Boil this mixture for a few minutes and add a few drops of honey. Now, consume it twice a day to strengthen your bones and get relief from your body ache.

Grape and Pectin Juice

Grapes are known for their high magnesium content, which is essential for our joints to function properly. Pectin, on the other hand, also provides relief to muscle pain. To start with, prepare a glass of freshly made grape juice and add a tablespoon of pectin mix in it. Stir it thoroughly and drink it once a day to strengthen your bones and muscles.

Dry Skin, Rashes, and Eczema

If you are suffering from any kind of problem related to your skin or hair, then you should definitely consider a natural treatment instead of an allopathic one. To start with, say goodbye to all those canned products and prefer having a gelatin-rich diet.

These days, having dry skins, rashes, pimples, or any other skin-related issues are quite common. Don't worry! With the help of these natural remedies, you can easily overcome it without any hassle.

Oils

Consider coconut oil, jojoba oil, and olive oil as your new best friends. If your skin rashes are mild, then you can go for either olive oil or coconut oil. Pour a few drops of oil to your palm and gently rub it on the infected area. If you are suffering from eczema, then prefer applying jojoba oil to the affected area for at least a week or two in order to get long-term results.

Honey and Butter Mix

This is a highly recommended solution to treat your dry skin and get immediate relief. To start with, take a few tablespoons of Shea butter and add the equal amount of honey to it. Also, add a few drops of lavender essential oil and stir the mixture thoroughly. Preserve it in an airtight container and use it multiple times a day.

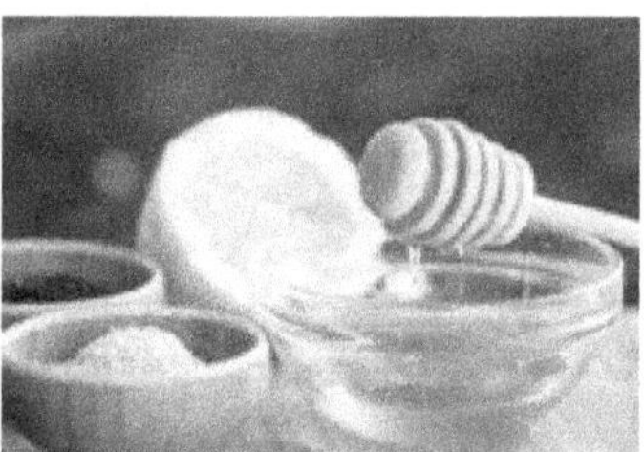

Baking Soda Bath

While oatmeal bath is considered as an excellent solution for burns and dry skin, you can also go for a baking soda bath to treat your skin-related issues. Simply prepare a cool bath and add a cup of baking soda in it. Stay in the bathtub for another 30 minutes at least to get rid of your skin impurities.

Apple Cider Vinegar

The multiple uses of apple cider vinegar can certainly surprise you. It can heal itchy and dry skin in no time. It is also an ideal treatment for poison ivy rashes as well. Just pour it into a container and with the help of cotton, apply it gently to the affected area. Though, you should make sure that it is only applicable for external usage.

Almond oil and Milk

Not just for external usage, you can also use almond oil to get rid of dry skin in different ways. Add 2-3 drops of almond oil in a glass of milk and drink it before going to bed. You will certainly see an evident difference in your skin in a matter of a few days.

Glycerin and Rose water

This is an ideal solution for chapped lips or dry skin. Simply pour some glycerin in a container and add an equal amount of rose water in it. Now, take a cotton bud and gently apply the solution to the infected area to get a soothing effect.

Mashed Banana and Honey

Too many times, due to change in weather, we suffer from dry skin. If you want to get a glowing skin in no time, then mash 2-3 bananas in a bowl and add a teaspoon of honey to the mixture. Now, apply this solution on your skin (even face) and get rid of any impurity. This can also help you get rid of pimples.

Now when you are familiar with different natural and homemade remedies for these common health issues, you can certainly ditch your medical bills and live a peaceful life. Move past those pills and give these alternative medical treatments a try to bring a much-needed change to your life.

Conclusion

I'm sure you must have had a great time reading this comprehensive guide about various naturopathy and alternative medical treatments. We have covered a wide range of solutions in this guide, so that you can find a cure to different health issues in a natural way.

While working on this guide, we walked an extra mile to make you familiar with various benefits of alternative treatments beforehand. Not only are these treatments cost-effective, but they won't cause any harmful side-effect to your body as well. With the assistance of these homemade natural remedies, you can say goodbye to all those pills and live a healthy lifestyle.

We have provided numerous natural remedies for a wide range of issues like headache, cold, flu, body pain, bad stomach, sore throat, and a lot more. To make things easier for you, we have listed an ideal way to prepare (and consume) these remedies. For every problem, we have listed multiple solutions, so that you can pick the one that appeals the most to you.

Go ahead and give these natural remedies a try. Don't experiment with your body by consuming all those biochemical pills. Take the right step and start treating your body like a temple.

Stay healthy and be safe!